LEAN

WEIGHT LOSS

HABITS

Stop Dieting, Lifelong Slimming, Better Eating,
Healthy Living, New Behaviors,
Don't Suffer & Stay Slim

JR FATE

Apex Book Publishing
www.apexbookpub.com

Contents

Introduction

So, you want to lose weight! Well, you are not alone. Except for a few fortunate people (who remain magically slim all their lives no matter what and how much they eat), a large part of the world needs to shed at least a few pounds. Weight loss, or more importantly, staying slim is one of the greatest challenges in today's age. There are plenty of distractions to keep you away from staying healthy and fit. Our lives have become mechanical, fast-paced, and insipid. We are slaves to our gadgets, erratic work schedules, and impulsive food habits.

We want to be healthy but we don't know the key to it. We don't know how to unlock the power to stay slim and healthy all our lives. Losing weight is easier in mind than in action for most of us. Nevertheless, if you have picked up this book and have sat down to read it, you have already begun your journey of living a holistically healthy life. So, congratulations!

Before you even begin thinking of ways to lose weight, remember to write a little note to yourself that says, "you are awesome!" You don't have to become like somebody else. If you get on the treadmill to transform yourself into some pinup model or a movie star, stop right there! That's not a good idea. Perhaps you are way better than those desirable bodies. So, love yourself. Think of your weight loss journey as a way of living a much happier and fulfilling life rather than getting into some meaningless envy game.

Staying slim is not a shallow idea as believed by many. Therefore, it should not be done for superficial reasons. You should not fall for quick fixes or crash diets. Starving doesn't make you look attractive. You should not look for quick weight loss diets or exercises. It has to be a constant in your life.

Being your ideal weight should reflect your holistic approach toward being your best in every possible way. The steps that you need to take to get that fit body are going to make you a more responsible and mindful individual. You will learn and practice being someone who's aware of their daily habits and choices. You will gain the power to change your mind, which will help you change your ways.

Begin with a mind shift to help you cultivate healthy habits in your everyday life, which will bring you long lasting results. As long as you focus on keeping a healthy mind, body, and soul, you will never gain an extra pound ever. You will stay slim naturally!

The goal of this book is to inspire you to look toward something that's more meaningful, sustainable, and rewarding in the long run.

CHAPTER 1

Mind Change Before Physical Change

Your mind is your best friend, and it can be your worst foe, too. It's up to you how you train your mind so that it gets the best of everything for you. There's nobody in the world who can rule, control, or change your thoughts. Each individual is the sole owner of their mind and thoughts, which is quite a power! Most of us don't take it very seriously and therefore, we don't understand the value of directing our mind to do the right thing for us.

A slim and healthy body is not something hard to maintain. In fact, that's the way we were born. Being physically fit should ideally be the norm. We have shifted to a mindset and a way of life that tells us to do whatever we feel like. Discipline is thrown out of the window. It's thought to be something boring or undesirable; something meant for only children or students. However, discipline simply means training your mind to do the right thing at the right time. Being disciplined doesn't mean being hard on yourself; it rather means to be kind to yourself because the outcome in the long run is going to be highly rewarding. Making up your mind about something and staying committed to it stems from discipline.

So let's get to the point—you want to get into a lean body and stay that way all your life. The key to getting a fit body is changing your mindset and developing the right habits. You cannot expect to see a physical change without a mind change. If your mind tells you to demolish a bar of chocolate anytime of the day, you probably have to deal with that first. You may sweat it out in the gym or go for a run, but the fat will come back because your mind is still the same. There's no harm in eating chocolates or that giant sized burger. However, they should not be in your thoughts. You should not eat anything just because there's nothing better to do. You can have "whatever" you like, but it should be eaten with the right mindset.

It's all about striking the right balance. You don't have to live to eat. You should eat to live. Your mind shouldn't control your actions. You should control your mind; and it happens with practice. You will need to create an atmosphere to be able to make a mind shift. Perhaps you will need to hang out with people who are disciplined about what they eat and their exercise routine.

Mind change is not so easy. You will have bursts of successes and a string of failures. But that's fine. As long as you are sincere about your goal of living in a healthy and lean body, you will achieve it sooner or later. Not everybody is the same. Everybody has different strengths of mind, different circumstances, and surroundings. Losing weight or staying slim can be harder for some people than others for various reasons—family, job, responsibilities, lifestyle, culture, lack of inspiration or motivation.

Whatever may be the case with you, just decide to treat your body well. Your friends, family, or spouse are not living in your body. It's you who is living in your body, so you need to take care of it, nurture it, and keep it healthy.

To see a physical change, you need a mind change, and here's how you do it –

Think on Purpose

Let your weight loss journey begin with your thoughts. Be intentional about what you think. If your mind wanders towards a pizza or a pasta, drag it back to salad. Keep thinking about eating healthy and staying healthy on purpose. The more you think that way, the more you will become that way.

People who you see are slim and super energetic think about staying that way. Their mind isn't able to entice them into eating anything on impulse.

Keep the End Goal in Mind

Visualize yourself as someone lean and fit. Keep the end result in mind while you work out or eat a nutritious meal. Don't think too much about how you appear now or how hard you have to work every day to lose weight. Most people fail at their weight loss plans because they get bored and tired of sticking to a routine.

After a while, they get back to their sweet comfort zone and procrastinate the idea of staying fit.

To keep at it, you need to remind yourself what you are going to achieve at the end of it—the happiness you will experience after you have shed those extra pounds and the freedom you will have to fit into any kind of clothes, the energy and the confidence that come along with it.

Develop Healthy Habits

Any habit whether it's good or bad stays with you forever, at least if you don't try hard to break it. Your habits are always by your side, giving you ample support in whatever you set your mind to. So why not have healthy habits? Decide to inculcate good daily habits that will help you march toward your weight loss goals. Don't give yourself any difficult targets. Start slow and easy. For instance, don't resolve to get up at 5 am every morning and go for a 10km run or eat no sugar whatsoever. Instead, give yourself mini challenges to build good habits, such as starting your day with a glass of water, doing a quick breathing exercise for five minutes, or cutting down on coffee.

Aim to develop one good habit every month and then build on it consistently. We all have heard that it takes at least 21 days to adapt to a habit. So, challenge yourself to stick to doing something for three weeks without fail—it could be going for a short walk, limiting sugar, spending more time outdoors, or sleeping early.

Live with Awareness

Being mindful of each action of yours is the key to living a great life. If you eat with awareness, go to bed and wake up with awareness, you will not be dismayed at what you see on the weighing scale. It's what you do each day that makes you who you are both from inside and outside. You can't depend on crash diets to become who you would like to be. Hunger is not the way to an ideal body weight. You don't deserve to starve yourself. You have got one life and you should be living it to the fullest.

Believe that being self-disciplined is a kind of self-care that leads to health, happiness, and peace.

Start Your Day Right

Mornings are the most beautiful time of the day. You have the opportunity to put everything behind and start afresh. Therefore, it's important to begin your day right (refer to the last chapter). There is no set rule to it, though. Each person can have their own way of starting their day. It could be with a prayer, reading something inspirational, going for a walk, listening to peaceful music, having a glass of water, or eating fresh fruits. Have your pick! The idea is to do something that helps you start the day on the right note.

There should be certain things you should refrain from doing as soon as you wake up, which can be checking your phone, work messages, smoking, having coffee or tea. Be particular about how you want to start your day and let that be something good.

Share Your Goals with Somebody

Talk about your goals with somebody you like or admire. Don't keep talking about it all the time, though. But make sure to share what you feel, think, and anticipate with at least one person. It's important to surround yourself with the right kind of people—the kind of people who understand the value of good health and good life. Don't spend too much time with people who have no inclination to stay fit. Of course, if your spouse or family are into eating unhealthy stuff and they have no intent to lose weight, it can be a challenging journey for you as well. In such a situation, you need to be even harder with your own self to realize your goals.

The objective of sharing your weight loss goals with somebody is to stay motivated and feel the energy to stay the course.

Write Down Your Goals

Writing down something on paper gives it more validity and assurance. Well, it's true. If you find it too hard to change your mindset about staying lean, try penning down your short-term targets. For instance, you can set a goal to lose two pounds in a week. Make a note of it in your diary and keep getting back to it. Remind yourself that you need to do it at any cost. After a week, get the weighing scale out and check if you have met the target. Keep it slow and progressive. It doesn't matter how slow your progress is, as long as you are moving in the right direction.

Give Accountability to Yourself

You should be answerable to your own self about your weight loss journey. It's a good idea to give accountability to somebody else as well. However, it's much better that you develop the mindset of staying committed and accountable about your fitness regime. For instance, if you have decided to avoid eating fat for dinner, then stop your hand from reaching out for the cheesecake on the table. You need to stay on your toes to be able to stay fit.

Yes of course, you can and you should indulge in your favorite dessert once in a while. That's not a bad idea at all. However, don't let that craving control your mind. Master the craving and enjoy it without guilt.

Reach Out to a Health Coach

You may want to get in touch with a health coach or a dietician for some advice on how to lose weight. Well, the idea is not to follow their advice to a tee, but just to help yourself slip into the mindset of eating well and getting fit. When you talk to a professional about something that you are trying to deal with, it has a greater influence on your mind. You get a chance to learn a lot of new things and it helps you get serious about the concerned matter. So, if it's fitness for you, talk to a fitness coach.

Spend Time Meditating

Meditation is the best way to set your mind on something. If you are trying to make a mind shift, change your habits, and adapt to a new lifestyle, spend some time meditating. Give yourself at least 10 to 30 minutes every day to just sit in a quiet place, in a relaxed position, and think about all that you want to do—eat nutritious food, exercise every day, take sunshine, sleep on time, and pursue a hobby. Don't think about what you want to give up (addictions or any bad habit). Just meditate upon what you want to do. Meditation is the most effective tool to strengthen your mind and thoughts about something.

Believe in Yourself

Don't feel like a loser just because you can't stick to a fitness regime. Remind yourself you are okay and there's nothing to feel bad about. Be it fitness or anything in life, it's important to stay strong and confident. Never compare yourself with anyone. You never know what health issues your slim and beautiful looking neighbor has. Everybody has their share of struggles and challenges. Nobody is perfect. Just believe in yourself that you can do whatever you decide to do.

Don’t Depend on Motivation

The biggest mistake that most people make is depending too much on motivation or inspiration. You should rather depend on routine to be able to do what you really want to do. If you want to wake up early, go to yoga class, eat healthy, stay active, and sleep at a particular time, set a routine for doing all of that. Don’t wait for the feeling of motivation or a sudden burst of mental energy to give you a kick to do what you are supposed to do. Motivation is not dependable. So why wait for it, anyway? You might feel super motivated a day and go for an hour walk and the motivation may continue for a day or two more, but after the third or fourth day, the motivation declines and you feel low in energy because you have not aligned your mind to a set routine.

When you have a fixed daily routine in place, you follow that no matter how you feel. The more you follow a routine, the easier it gets to start liking it eventually. Motivation or no motivation, just do what you need to do.

Read Quite a Few Fitness Books

What you read leaves an impression on your mind. Pick up a good health, diet, or fitness book and read it from cover to cover. Yes, you are reading one right now. So, you have already tickled your mind to think differently and make fitness an integral part of life. Reading about sensible weight loss and healthy lifestyle will help you incorporate fitness in your daily life. For instance, you may not like having fruits much, but after knowing their benefits and how they aid in weight loss, you might just start having a fruit bowl every morning.

As your mind begins to shift toward making you develop good daily habits, focusing on self-care, being mindful, and making progress, you will soon realize that maintaining an ideal body weight is a norm with you.

CHAPTER 2

Watch Out for the Boomerang Effect

Don't shed weight just to get it all back! The wrong way of losing weight is going to do your body more harm than good. So be careful how you slim down. The usual mindset wants to lose extra body fat as fast as possible. People go on fad diets to be able to look a certain way within a short time frame for a certain occasion. Why make yourself suffer just to fit into an outfit and then get back to being worse?

Quick weight loss will not work in the long run of life. Just understand and accept it. You cannot be your desired weight in a fast or easy way. Remember, fast weight loss means fast weight gain. The popular phenomenon known as the boomerang effect is about how the majority of people lose weight only to get it back. Most people don't understand that weight loss should be a slow and constant process.

So, what happens when your body loses a lot of weight in a short span of time? Let's understand this—weight loss affects our body organs. Our hormones respond in a different way after we have shed some pounds quickly. The metabolism slows down and you are unable to lose many calories because of the imbalance in the energy equation; the feeling of fullness and satiety decline. You feel hungry quite soon and you want to fill your belly more than it's required.

Weight loss doesn't always mean fat loss. With an erroneous diet, you simply lose muscle mass and the fat remains where it was. Besides, fast weight loss diets make your body miss out on vital nutrients, which leads to fatigue, hair loss, low immunity, and various other health problems.

Fast weight loss may take you on a high for some time, while it lasts. However, once you get back to your old habits and lifestyle, the boomerang effect is a bit too much to deal with. The secret to staying slim all your life is quite simple—do it slow so that it becomes a habit. We need to make weight maintenance a habit. There's no magic potion to it.

So, think about your real goals before you even consider any crazy diet plan. What do you really want in terms of your body and health? You should think long-term, even though it's hard. You may have to wait longer to get thin, but it will sustain.

Negative Effects of Fast Weight Loss

You Gain Weight Faster

The most adverse effect of fast weight loss is that you gain weight again way faster. Your body hasn't got used to eating less. Your mind is not aligned to exercising regularly. The diet plan you followed probably took away a lot of your mental and physical energy. Now you feel more lethargic, hungrier, and more depressed because the results haven't lasted long. You begin to see more fat in your body—because you are eating way more than you used to eat.

Your Body Organs Suffer

Your body doesn't respond well to quick weight loss. It feels dehydrated because the weight loss that you experience is actually water that you lose and not fat. That happens because when you take limited or no carbohydrates, the primary source of energy that your body burns is glycogen—it's a type of carbohydrate stored in your liver and muscles, and 3 grams of water are affixed to every gram of carbohydrate in your body. Thus, when you utilize all your glycogen, the adjacent water exits the body. Fast weight loss diets make people lose so much water that they get dehydrated.

You Feel More Demotivated and Out of Energy

When you get the same (or more) weight back in your body, you will obviously feel demotivated and out of energy. The quick shift to a lighter body doesn't work because your mind takes its own time to adjust to changes. You can't discipline your body for a few days and expect it to give you lifelong results. If you are hard on your body—not giving it a wholesome diet because you want to shed a few pounds fast, your body will get into a revenge mode and demand more food.

It Impacts Your Mental Health

Gaining more weight after a sudden weight loss is not good for your mental health as well. You feel a sense of loss, a feeling of failure weighs you down. The real victory is in keeping an ideal weight maintained by adapting to a sensible weight loss regime.

However, when you lose weight only for a short while just to get it all back, it makes you feel depressed and you feel like eating more even when you are not hungry.

It Gets Tougher to Lose Weight Again

Of course, it becomes even harder to lose weight after you have gained it back. It will require you to have a much higher level of will power and discipline to get on the treadmill and a good diet plan all over again. You can eventually lose weight with a healthy diet plan and exercise regime, but your body and mind will take time to adjust to it.

How to Get Rid of 'Quick Weight Loss' Mentality

Think Long-Term

The best way to get rid of this mentality of fast weight loss is to have a long-term view of your health. Aim to lose weight not just to look good but to feel good as well. Read good health books, talk to professionals, and learn from real-life examples—

understand how good health is beneficial in the long run. Try to develop a mature perspective about staying slim.

When you have a long-term view of fitness, you will automatically make better decisions in regards to what you eat. You will become a sensible eater without much struggle. As you keep pressing on, you will get into the habit of eating right no matter what the situation is—whether you are alone with nothing to eat or at a party with tons of options to choose from.

Learn About Your Body

Be aware of your body, know what it needs. Understand that your body needs nutrients to function properly. Don't deny your body of carbs. The food that you have been eating for ages (the food that your grandparents have been feeding your parents, and your parents have been feeding you) is meant to give strength to your body. Thus, when you deny your body the traditional good food, it doesn't work very well in the long run. In fact, you should deny yourself modern-age food, which is low in nutrition but high in calories.

Apart from food, your body also needs rest and relaxation. So give your body sufficient food. Don't overeat or starve. Moderation is the key to achieving a lean body. You can enjoy your favorite bread, but there's a difference between having a slice and having a loaf.

Consider Your Gender, Age, and Environment

You should understand that diet plans and exercises are different for different people according to their gender, age and the kind of environment they live in. There are people who are into jobs that require a lot of physical labor like athletes, dancers, nurses, or technicians. They need more food than those who do less physical activity, such as call center operators, accountants, and receptionists. Then you should consider your age and gender—as you advance in years, you should be eating less considering the amount of physical exercise you can do.

Prioritize Health Over Weight

Lastly, it's important to prioritize your health over your weight. You may weigh a pound or two extra but as long as you are healthy from within, it should not bother you. You should focus on staying lean with an idea of staying active and energetic. A healthy body is about a lot of things—strong immune system, good digestive system, energy, and the functionality of organs. Besides, it's also about your mental, spiritual, and social wellbeing. A slim body is something you can easily achieve and sustain when you take care of your overall health.

Don't go for fast weight loss diets. They are not sustainable. To lose weight and stay lean all your life, have a broader perspective about weight loss and health.

CHAPTER 3

How Much Should You Eat

Eating right should be a habit to keep your weight in check. So how much should you eat to stay slim? Should you really count calories or weigh what you eat? Well, the basic idea of eating right is to know what you are eating. Eat with awareness. Most of the time we don't realize what we are putting in our mouths. We end up eating stuff that's low in nutrition and high in everything unhealthy. That happens when we are hungry or just bored. To avoid that, make sure you follow a set timetable of taking your meals.

Make sure your diet has enough nutrients for your body—most of your food should have vitamins, fiber, minerals, and other nutrients. You should have lots of fresh fruits and vegetables, lean protein, low-fat dairy, and whole grains. You should restrict the consumption of added sugar, solid fats, and sodium.

When you eat right, you naturally feel more energetic and happy. So, let's get down to understanding the right food choices—

Carbs, Fat, and Calories

While some people are totally unaware of what they are eating, some like to count every calorie they take in. Don't overstress yourself by counting calories or carbs. The better approach is to eat in moderation and to take care of the portion size. Instead of not eating something at all, you should eat it less. For instance, if you are fond of rice, eat it in a certain proportion to other things. Eat more veggies with a smaller portion of rice.

Carbs Are Not Bad

Most people who want to lose weight choose to eat low or zero carbohydrates. But that's not the right thing to do. Remember, carbs give us energy. Before you discard something from your diet, understand why you are doing so. Don't just stop eating something foundational because that's the trend. Yes, you are able to lose a lot of weight with reduced carb intake. However, that takes a lot away from your body. Carbs are a combination of fiber, starch, and sugars.

Instead of lowering or not eating any carbs at all, choose the right carbs for your body. Do a little bit of research on the nutritional value of different foods that you enjoy eating, read the nutrition labels on various products that you buy. Your carbs intake should depend on how much your body needs it. Also, not all carbs are bad. Yes, you should limit the intake of refined carbs, such as white flour, refined grains, and refined sugars. In fact, it's better you don't take them at all if you come under a certain age bracket (40 and above). However, if you eat complex carbs, such as whole grain breads and cereals, oats, corn, legumes, and fiber-rich fruits and vegetables, you will be able to maintain a healthy weight quite naturally.

Choose Your Fats Carefully

Fat is not your best buddy when you want to lose weight. Fat makes you "fat" and gives you high cholesterol, which is not good for your health. However, fat also protects your heart if the right kind of fats are taken in the right measure. There are different types of fats, such as saturated fat, trans fat, unsaturated fat, monounsaturated fat, and polyunsaturated fat. Each kind of fat has a role to play when we eat them. It's up to us how much we eat them to take the benefit out of them or simply gain weight.

- Saturated fat is found mostly in animal foods, such as pork, beef, lamb, whole milk, butter, some tropical oils, and baked eatables. You should not eat much saturated fat as too much saturated fat increases the bad cholesterol levels (LDL) in your blood.
- Trans fat is found in most of the packaged food stuff that we buy, such as coffee cream, cakes, cookies, shortening, and solid margarine. Trans fat intake should ideally be zero as it increases the bad cholesterol and decreases the good cholesterol (HDL).
- Unsaturated fat—monounsaturated and polyunsaturated fat. The two types of fat are considered to be good fat, as it helps in keeping your cholesterol levels in check. They raise the level of good cholesterol in your blood. The unsaturated fat is found in plant-based foods, such as nuts, seeds, olives, canola, peanut oils, avocado, walnuts, flax seeds, and soybeans. So, you should consume such fat quite regularly.

Cut Down on Added Sugars and Sodium

Although taking added sugar in low quantities isn't particularly harmful, it has no nutritional value. Added sugar is empty calories. When you eat food items like sugary drinks, candy, desserts, ice creams, and chocolates, your blood sugar level increases giving a boost to your blood insulin, which causes you to feel low in energy after a while. The instant energy that you feel as soon as you take refined sugar doesn't last long.

You should rather have plenty of water, fresh fruit juices, and all kinds of water-rich foods like cucumbers and lemons to feel energetic all the time.

Similarly, you should not take too much of sodium, which is refined salt, in your diet. Your body needs only a small amount of sodium to function properly. A high intake of sodium can give you high blood pressure and other diseases. You should avoid food stuff like pizzas, tacos, sandwiches, savory snacks, and burgers to limit your sodium intake.

You should switch to healthier alternatives like seasonings of herbs and spices to add pungency in your meals.

Get a Food Scale and Start Weighing the Food You Eat

Well, weighing your food may not be everyone's cup of tea. It may feel like a bit too much of an effort. Who wants to be so particular about counting each calorie? Yes, it may be a bit too much of a fixation with weight loss. As long as you can manage portion control on your own, nothing like it. Some of you might be able to do it without a food scale, which is great. However, many of you will not be able to keep your appetite in check and you will end up eating more than you are supposed to.

If you are serious about your weight loss, you need to be mindful of how many calories you consume in a day. You need to make sure that you don't consume more calories than you need for a day. The idea of weighing food is to help you control portions and shed extra pounds in a sustainable way and keep them off.

When you start with a new diet plan, your food scale can actually teach you about correct serving sizes. You will soon realize that the portion you thought was four ounces is actually eight ounces. Such a mistake could hamper your diet. And, you don't want that, right? You don't have to measure your food all your life. It's just for the time period when you are trying hard to be your ideal weight. After a while, you will begin to understand different portion sizes of different foods that you typically eat and you will naturally choose the right serving size.

Alternatively, you can also use your plate as a portion control guide:

- High-quality protein, such as fish, eggs, meat, beans, and dairy should be a quarter of a plate.
- Vegetables and salads should be half a plate.

- Complex carbs, such as starchy vegetables and whole grains should be quarter of a plate.
- High-fat foods, such as cheese, butter, and oil should be half a tablespoon.

The above guide can vary based on a person's dietary needs. People who are physically active can increase the portion size.

You can easily get into the habit of portion control at home. But what about restaurant visits and social gatherings? How would you control what you eat without annoying anyone? Well, you need to be a little clever in such situations and manage to eat less without making a big deal about it. At a restaurant, you can order half a portion of a dish if possible, or share a full portion with someone. You can also just satiate your appetite with some healthy starters and not have the main course.

A few other effective ways of portion control:

- Drink a glass of water half an hour before every meal. It will reduce your chances of overeating.
- Try to eat slowly. You are more likely to overeat when you eat fast because your brain can take some time to realize that you have eaten enough. So, give it some time and enjoy your food at a leisurely pace.
- Trick your mind by eating in small plates or bowls. When you take a small plate to eat, you will automatically eat less.

- You can also keep a food diary or log your meals in a food journaling app. Jotting down how much you eat can also help you stay on track.

The basic cause of gaining extra weight is overeating. Therefore, it's important to deal with the root cause first before you incorporate other things in your lifestyle.

Start a Routine of Intermittent Fasting

Intermittent fasting is quite a popular idea these days adopted by many for healthy weight loss and gut cleaning. It's also considered to be beneficial for curing a lot of common diseases, such as diabetes, blood pressure, and cholesterol. When you go without food for a certain number of hours, your stomach gets a chance to rest and the intestines get cleaned up in the process, which eventually aids in blood purification. The idea is that diseases cannot exist in a clean body.

Let's understand how intermittent fasting helps in weight loss. When you fast for a certain number of hours in a day, your insulin levels decrease and your fat cells are then able to release their stored sugar, to be used as energy. You lose weight when you allow your insulin levels to go down for a long period of time so that the stored fat in your body gets a chance to be used and burn off.

The food you eat is broken down by enzymes in your gut and eventually turns into molecules in your bloodstream. Refined carbohydrates, such as white flour and white rice readily convert into sugar, which your cells use for energy. If your cells don't use it all, you store it as fat. However, sugar can only seep into our cells with insulin, a hormone produced in the pancreas. Insulin directs sugar into the fat cells and keeps it stored there.

How to Fast Intermittently

The most basic idea of intermittent fasting is to go without food for straight 16 hours and eat only within the window of eight hours. So it works like this—if you have your first meal at 10 am, your last meal has to be at 6 pm, after which you are not supposed to eat anything. For instance, if you'd like to have dinner at 7 pm, then have your breakfast at 11 am. It might not be so easy to adapt to initially, as you might feel hungry way past your dinner time (if you stay awake till 11 or 12 pm). You should ideally be asleep by 9 - 9:30 pm after you have had dinner at 7 pm. So your sleep pattern also makes a difference in how well you can adapt to the routine of intermittent fasting.

If you follow a routine and sleep on a set time, eating for eight hours and fasting for 16 hours is not going to be too hard. You need to keep in mind that you will be sleeping most of the time while you are fasting. Besides, you can have zero-calorie beverages, such as water, black tea or coffee during your fast to help you feel less stressed about not eating.

There are other ways of intermittent fasting, such as taking all your meals normally five days a week and taking only 500-600 calories a day for the remaining two days. You can also fast alternate days or once a week. However, fasting doesn't mean that you can eat whatever you feel like during your eating window. To lose weight healthily, you need to eat only nutritious food and stay away from all sorts of junk food.

Is Intermittent Fasting Safe

Intermittent fasting may not be for everyone. While some people are able to take substantial health benefits out of it, some are unable to cope with it. If you have never fasted in your life, you should first consult your doctor before choosing any method of intermittent fasting.

You should not fast if you:

- Are pregnant
- Are a breastfeeding mother
- Have a medical condition
- Are below the age of 18
- Have a history of eating disorders

Studies and research indicate that intermittent fasting is safe for most people. However, you should do it in the right way. There are certain things you should keep in mind to be able to reap maximum benefit out of it:

- Replace your unhealthy snacks (potato chips, pretzels, cakes and cookies) with fruits and vegetables, lean proteins (plain yogurt, cottage cheese, beans, legumes, chicken, eggs, and quinoa), and healthy fats (avocado, fatty fish, chia seeds, and all sorts of nuts).

- Allow your body to burn fat between meals. Stay active through the day.
- Try an easy method of intermittent fasting—limit the hours of eating. For instance, you can squeeze all your meals between 7 a.m. to 3 p.m. The earlier it is, the better. Don't choose hours of eating toward bed time.
- Refrain from eating or snacking at night.

Benefits of Long-Term Intermittent Fasting

- The first benefit you want to talk about is weight loss, which you can see after a few weeks or months depending on factors like age, gender, metabolism, weight history, and overall lifestyle of a person. Studies suggest that a lot of obese men are able to lose a lot of fat as they practice intermittent fasting.
- Since intermittent fasting aids in gut cleaning, a lot of diseases are reversed. It improves your blood pressure and heart health.
- Intermittent fasting helps in reducing cell damages that occur due to inflammation and oxidation.
- Fasting lowers blood sugar level, which reduces the risk of diabetes.
- When you stop snacking unnecessarily, the stored fat in your body is used as energy, which helps in reducing belly fat.
- Intermittent fasting lowers the risk of cancer.

Conscious eating leads to healthy and long-term weight loss. Weighing your food, keeping a check on portions, and fasting can change your idea about food. You will understand that food is necessary for survival, but it should not have adverse effects on your health.

CHAPTER 4

Get Up and Get Going

Staying active is the secret to being slim. Walking may seem like something very simple, but it can be a game changer in many ways. Let's begin with the simplest of facts that the more you walk, the more calories you burn. Even though we know the benefits of walking and staying active, we don't walk as much as we should. We know the medicine of good life, but we choose to sit around and be lazy.

Walking is, undoubtedly, the easiest workout regime for anybody of any age group. Even if you have never exercised in your life, you can still walk! You don't need a very flexible body to be able to walk. Most of us have excuses for not walking enough—it could be busy work schedules, household chores, other distractions, or just lack of inclination. The unfortunate part is that we miss out on so many benefits that result from just moving our limbs.

Instead of making excuses for not being able to walk, you should rather look out for opportunities to walk as much as possible. If you want to be lean, energetic, and healthy from within, walking should be an integral part of your lifestyle. Besides, giving it a dedicated time, you should stand more and stop sitting around for long hours. If your job requires you to sit for hours, make it a point to stand up for at least three minutes every 30 minutes.

The idea is not to wait for that "half an hour" when you will go for a walk. That may never happen. Before you get to that level of discipline, give yourself small opportunities of physical activities throughout the day. Perhaps you can park your car a little farther away so that you can walk a little more; you can go to the office pantry for a refill of water, run a short errand for a colleague, or simply stand by a window for five minutes after lunch.

Walk As Much As You Can

If you are someone who's just not able to stick to a walk schedule, you are not alone. We all procrastinate on our walks and then we go on a guilt trip and come back with two scoops of our favorite chocolate chip ice cream. Well, stop feeling grouchy about it. Instead of giving yourself big targets, be determined about moving around in small bits.

Don't be a procrastinator! Just do it!

Walk to the Grocery Store

Give yourself some physical retail therapy. Try and limit ordering groceries online. The more we rely on technology, the lazier we become. Instead of ordering every single thing online, make it a point to pick a few things up yourself by visiting a grocery store. Do it just to drag yourself out of the house and get on your feet.

Take the Stairs

The easiest way to shake off a few calories is by taking the stairs instead of the elevator. Be it your home or office, it's no joy waiting for the elevator to arrive and then realize you have reached the wrong floor or worse the underground parking instead of the floor you wanted to go to. Enjoy climbing the stairs, burn some fat, and feel good about yourself.

Stand in the Queue

Although it's not fun to wait in a queue for anything, it can be one of your moments to stretch your body a little bit. Begin to like queues because they give you a chance to stand for a while, which is better than sitting for long hours. Next time you stand in a queue, remember to enjoy it.

Stand Up at Work

Try to stand up at work whenever possible. If there's a quick team huddle, stand and talk to your team. Besides, you can stand up once in a while even when there's nobody around to talk to, just to remind yourself that you have been sitting for quite some time.

Do a Bit of Cleaning Every Day

Whether you are at home or work, get down to doing a bit of cleaning every day. You can clean your desk, declutter your drawers, or simply clear the wastepaper basket. The idea is to move around a bit, get going, and stay active.

Do a Bit of Stretching at Your Desk

You can do a bit of exercise and stretching at your desk while at work. You don't have to feel shy because that's necessary for you. And, who knows? You might inspire your colleagues to join you for a quick workout session.

Go For a Lunch Break Walk

Post-lunch office hours are a bit snoozy. Thus, you should utilize your lunch break as an opportunity to walk around and feel refreshed. You can either time your walk or just walk as much as you can till you see everybody is back to their desks. Even if you get to walk for ten minutes, it can take your energy levels up.

Find Excuses to Chit-Chat with Colleagues

You should walk up to your colleagues once or twice a day to have a quick chit-chat or maybe grab a coffee together. It's definitely one of the ways to keep yourself mentally and physically energetic throughout the day.

Walk While You Talk on Phone

Everybody gets to spend at least some time on their phone every once in a while. Take the opportunity to walk as you talk on the phone. Go out to breathe in some fresh air as well while you are talking. Although the use of gadgets should be limited, we can use them to our benefit sometimes.

Track Your Steps

Your phone probably should have a default app that tracks your steps throughout the day. You can use it to keep a track of how much you walked in a day. It will keep you motivated as you will see the number of steps walked. You can challenge yourself to keep increasing the number of steps taken in a day.

Miss the Bus

It's a good idea to miss the bus sometimes and walk a mile or two. While you may not want to do it every day, it can be one of the ways to walk more. You can even make it more fun by increasing the number of miles you walk. From a couple of miles, you can increase it to five miles or more, which will help you increase your level of stamina and energy to walk.

How To Develop the Habit of Regular Walks

After you have trained your mind about staying active throughout the day, you can slowly get into a serious walk regime. You should start going for walks either in the mornings or evenings, whenever you can manage your time. The basic idea to keep in mind is that you will never get time to walk. No matter how hard you try, you will always be running short of time. Therefore, you will have to manage your time to be able to keep at least half an hour aside for a dedicated walk time.

Start with some warmup exercises like stretching, arm circles, and leg swings. If you have never walked or been part of any physical activity in a long time, take it easy. Walk for only 10-15 minutes in the beginning. Besides, it's advisable to consider your age and overall health before you begin with a new exercise regime.

For a normal healthy individual, a minimum of 30 minutes of brisk walk every day is the most basic physical workout. So, get going!

Prepare Your Mind

To start with a regular walk regime, you should make up your mind about it. Don't be casual or random about your walks. Decide in advance if you want to go for a walk five times a week, four times a week, or thrice a week. If it's well planned and thought out in your mind, you will find it much easier to stay motivated about it.

Create an Atmosphere

Keep your track pants, t-shirt, and running shoes ready right next to your bed, so that you see them the first thing as soon as you wake up. Set the alarm, keep the watch by your side (a little away so that you need to get up to put it off), and go to sleep on time. Give yourself sufficient hours to sleep so that you are able to get up without struggle.

Take Help of a Fitness App

Download a good fitness app on your phone to help you stay on track with your walks. You can track your footsteps or the number of calories burned in a specific period of time. There has to be something to focus on to keep going. Although you can walk for as much time as you want, keeping a track of your progress via an app is always more helpful.

Give Yourself Certain Goals

You will enjoy your walks more when you make them goal driven. You can set different types of goals and targets, such as walking for half an hour every day for a week or running for at least 10 minutes five times a week. You can also aim to lose certain pounds in a span of 15 days. However, focusing too much on tracking the pounds shed is not a good idea. Just focus on walking as much as possible and try staying consistent with it.

Increase Your Level Slowly

Start with walking for 20 minutes every day. Push yourself slowly toward walking more and more as you learn to be consistent. For instance, keep walking for 20 minutes for the first week, and then increase your level up to 30 minutes, and eventually 45 minutes to an hour.

Push Yourself When You Need To

You will feel like not going for a walk quite often until it becomes a habit. Remember, it takes a while to make an activity your habit. So, you will need to push yourself real hard at times to keep at it. You can take a break from walking, but it should not be very long. When you begin again, you will have to work at it from scratch. Going for a walk every day is an investment that you make toward your health. Therefore, it's important to be regular to be able to see some reward. If you break the regularity, it's much harder to get back to it.

Look for Alternatives

If you don't feel like going for a walk, think of some other physical activity that you like. It could be dancing, swimming, or playing an outdoor sport. Do what you enjoy the most and stick to it.

Get Creative

It's important to enjoy your walks and you should look forward to it every day. It should not feel like a task, which is why you should incorporate some change and creativity into your workout regime. For instance, you can choose to go to a new park or a beach instead of the one that you usually go to.

Listen to Some Good Music or Podcast

The best way to prolong your walks or workout sessions is to listen to some real good music or a podcast. Keep your playlist ready as you set out for a walk and let your favorite tunes make you sweat it all out. It's quite easy to walk for long while listening to something interesting.

Invite a Walk Buddy

If you have gotten bored walking alone, you can invite somebody to come with you for walks. When two people walk or work out together, there's an intuitive competitiveness between them that keeps them both on track. You can also join a group of fitness freaks to keep yourself elevated about staying fit.

Benefits of Walking

Besides the obvious benefit of weight loss, walking has many other benefits that we should be aware of. Staying active does not just keep you physically fit, but it also helps you stay mentally and emotionally happy. Therefore, the more you walk the better it is.

Helps You Maintain Your Ideal Body Weight

Needless to say, you can maintain your desired body weight by just walking every day. It's up to you how many times you want to go for a walk in a week and for how long you want to walk, but the result is a lean and fit body. Walking is the easiest way to burn calories and keeps you from gaining any extra weight. Yes of course, if you overeat, you will need to sweat it out more to be able to shed off extra calories.

Reduces Your Belly Fat

Walking can keep your belly tucked in. Most people are able to lose a few inches off their waistlines by simply walking regularly. According to studies, men with a waistline of over 40 inches and women with more than 35 inches are more likely to have heart disease and type 2 diabetes. Besides, who likes to have extra flab hanging around their waist? It's possible to get rid of it by walking for at least 60 minutes a day, three to four times a week.

Makes You Physically Stronger

Walking can make your bones and joints stronger. It also helps in making your muscles look more toned and nice. People who follow a consistent walk routine have stronger stamina than those who do not walk.

Keeps Diseases Away

As mentioned earlier, you can keep a lot of diseases at bay with a regular walking routine. Walking keeps your body in function, makes all your organs more active and diseases have no chance taking any form in your body. A physically active lifestyle can keep your body safe from diseases like heart disease, stroke, diabetes, blood pressure, high cholesterol, and joint and muscular pain.

Builds a Good Immune System

Walking and exercising can also build your immune system. When you live a sedentary life, whatever you eat doesn't get utilized by your body very well. Even if you eat nutritious food, your body needs to move around to be able to absorb nutrients properly. The more you sit, the more lethargic you become and your body kind of stops responding to anything the way it should, which affects your immunity.

A good immune system is a combination of physical activeness, good food, sunshine, fresh air, and sufficient sleep.

Good For Heart and Lung Fitness

When you walk at a certain pace, your heart and lungs are in use because they work toward supplying oxygen to your muscles. You breathe more consciously, which helps in improving your heart and lung health. As you get used to walking and exercising every day, your body becomes more efficacious at getting oxygen into the bloodstream and supplying it to the functioning muscles. You will realize that shortness of breath has decreased over time.

Improves Your Thinking Ability

When you walk or get into any kind of physical activity, the blood flow increases, which also helps in improving your thinking ability. The key to overall good functioning of your body and brain is the proper blood circulation, which is achieved by standing on your two feet and walking.

Remember, your brain uses about 20% of your body's total oxygen supply, so if you are not receiving sufficient oxygen up there, it's easy to lose focus. You must have noticed that you feel more refreshed, and you get new ideas after you come back from a walk.

Uplifts Your Mood

Walking is not just an exercise, but it's your excuse to have your own time alone. It helps you connect with your own self, which most of us don't care about. When you walk, your whole body, mind, heart, and soul come together. You feel a sense of freedom and abandonment, which automatically raises your spirits and makes you feel good. It's an effective way to combat stress and anxiety.

If you do not walk as regularly as you should, make it an integral part of your life. It's never too late. You can start today.

CHAPTER 5

Get Better Sleep

There's a reason why your body needs to rest. Not just your body, but your mind also needs to rest to be able to refresh, recharge, and renew. While some people sleep for longer hours, there are people who are often sleep deprived. There are some unconventional ideologies associated with sleep that say we don't need to sleep too much—sleeping for five hours is enough. Well, different experts will have different viewpoints. The right approach is to be disciplined about your sleep. Neither should you sleep less nor should you sleep more. Just like all other aspects of your well-being, you need to have a balanced approach toward your sleep as well.

Sleep is vital to our being. We cannot function without getting sufficient sleep. So how much should you sleep to be able to function properly and stay healthy? According to studies, the number of hours you need to sleep largely depends on your age. If you are a young adult, you need to sleep for seven to nine hours. People older than the age of 65 should sleep for seven to eight hours. So, the rough estimate is that an eight hour sleep is good enough for most of us.

How Does Sleep Help in Maintaining Your Body Weight?

Going to bed can make a huge difference to your physical fitness and body weight. When you sleep, your hunger hormones are also at rest. Ghrelin, a hormone that stimulates appetite, declines while you are sleeping. However, when you are awake ghrelin increases, and another hormone called leptin that makes you feel satiated after eating decreases—the imbalance makes you feel hungry.

Research indicates that lack of sleep can lead to health issues like obesity, type 2 diabetes, and metabolic syndrome.

When you are awake while you are supposed to sleep, your brain automatically nudges you to snack on something for the sake of it. You get this false illusion that you are hungry and then you end up eating anything that you get your hands on.

Therefore, it's essential to follow a sleep routine every night. Most people make the mistake of going to bed at random times—sometimes at 11 pm while sometimes it's 12:30 am or even later. The time you want to wake up is hugely dependent on what time you go to sleep. So, set a proper bedtime and stick to it no matter what.

How to Create a Sleep Routine

A sleep routine is an important part of following a healthy lifestyle. If you want to stay fit physically, mentally, and emotionally, make it a point to go to sleep at a fixed time every night. Don't take your sleep time for granted. If it's 10 o'clock, keep it that way as long as you can control it. Of course, there are occasions when it's totally impractical to follow a sleep routine, such as vacations, night outs, or get-togethers. In such situations, you can prolong your time to stay awake. However, that should not be too often. Breaking your routine should be a rare thing.

Decide a Bedtime and Stick To It

Make up your mind about when you want to go to bed every night. The earlier you go to sleep, the better it is. If you go to sleep early, you will naturally get into the habit of waking up early, too. For instance, if you sleep for eight hours and you decide to sleep at 10:30 pm every night, you will wake up fresh by 6:30 am, which is a good practice.

Sleeping on a set time can be developed into a habit by sticking to it for a long time. You might have to push yourself a bit too hard initially. For instance, you will have to follow the routine even on the weekends to be able to stay consistent.

Plan Your Dinner Time Accordingly

Your dinner time has to be at least two hours before your bedtime. If you are going to sleep at 10 pm, make sure you have had dinner by 8 pm. If you choose to sleep early at around 9:30 pm, then have your dinner at 7 or 7:30 pm. Don't have large meals just around the bedtime. In fact, it's better to have something light for dinner, such as soups or sauteed veggies.

Keep Distractions Away

The biggest bedtime challenge to combat is the different distractions, such as your gadgets, TV, or your children playing around (it's a good idea to put your children to sleep before you go to sleep). Put your phone, tab, and laptop away. Being glued to your gadgets affects the quality of your sleep. Your bedroom should be a place for rest and relaxation. Try to keep everything else away, apart from what's needed in a place to sleep.

Create a Comfortable Sleep Atmosphere

Make sure your pillows, mattress, and blankets are comfortable. The lights should be off or dim. The room temperature should be moderate. A calm environment can help you fall asleep with ease. Besides, you will have to make sure the person who sleeps with you follows the same sleep routine. For instance, if your spouse likes to watch a movie before dozing off, you might have to deal with it. While some people are able to fall asleep even with distractions around, there are people who need absolute silence.

Get Into the Mood of Sleeping

It's important to get into the mood of retiring to bed. Change into your night clothes. Don't plan to go out, watch a movie, or play a game around your sleep time. You will be cajoled by people around to be up for some activity, but you should be particular about your sleep routine.

If you like to read a book before you fall asleep, you can do that. However, it's advisable to read something positive before you shut your eyes.

Abstain From Coffee or Tea Toward Bedtime

Some people like the idea of having a nightcap. However, it may hamper your sleep. So, avoid caffeine or any kind of beverage just before bed. Let your body and mind know it's time to sleep. Just keep a water jar by your bedside so that you don't have to get up and go to the kitchen when you get thirsty in the middle of night.

Stay Active Throughout the Day

To be able to fall asleep at your set time, you should try to stay active throughout the day. Being busy with different things during the day helps you get into the rest mode quite naturally. Your body demands rest and relaxation at the end of a tiring day. So, make sure you spend your days constructively and accomplish quite a few things.

Avoid Long Afternoon Naps

Some people like to enjoy afternoon naps post lunch, which is not bad at all. Of course, if you need to go to work, you don't have that privilege. However, even if you do take afternoon naps, make sure they are not too long. Taking a midday nap for fifteen minutes to half an hour is good enough. If you sleep longer during the day, you might not feel too sleepy around the bedtime.

Let Everybody Around Know About Your Bedtime

Make sure your folks at home are aware of your sleep time and they don't disturb you around that time. There's no point trying to sleep while everybody else around expects you to be awake. It's better to announce your sleep routine to your family so that they leave you alone, or they might also follow in your footsteps.

Benefits of a Good Night's Sleep

A good night's sleep is as important as a well balanced diet. If you eat well and exercise, but you don't sleep properly, you will miss out on many health benefits. To live a holistically rewarding life, sleeping on time and for a sufficient number of hours are necessary.

Sharpens Your Brain

When you sleep, your brain also takes rest. That's when it gets time to renew and refresh just like your other body organs. If you are sleep deprived, your brain doesn't work as sharp as it's supposed to be, because it's fatigued. People who get sufficient and undisturbed sleep every night are more alert and active throughout the day. They are able to focus better on whatever they are supposed to do for a living. Sleep improves concentration and productivity.

Good For Your Emotional Well-Being

A good night's sleep helps you stay happy and satisfied. You are less irritable or cranky during the day. When you don't get to sleep properly for a prolonged period of time, it affects your emotions. Sleep helps you handle stress better, as it gives you time to heal and restore. It takes care of your mood and feelings—refreshes you and helps you think from a new perspective as you wake up.

Boosts Your Immune System

Sleep has a vital role to play in your body's immune system. When your body is in rest mode, your immune cells and proteins get the rest they require to guard against all sorts of germs. Taking high-quality sleep for a sufficient number of hours at night enables your body to develop a well-balanced immune defense that comprises innate and adaptive immunity.

Good For Your Heart

Sleep protects your heart, too. According to studies, a person who's sleep deprived has more chances of calcium buildup in their heart's arteries. Apparently, people who sleep less than six hours per night are at a higher risk of developing changes in the arteries of the heart. Sleeping well helps your heart rate stay normal and you feel more relaxed, which aids in keeping your blood pressure in control.

Keeps Your Body Weight Stable

Lack of sleep decreases your body's production of certain appetite-controlling hormones, which may lead to weight gain. Several studies indicate that not getting enough sleep raises ghrelin and reduces leptin (hormones that keep your metabolism in check), compared with those who slept for seven to eight hours at night. Not going to bed on time makes you binge on snacks, which hinders your weight management.

While sleep is an integral part of your well-being, sleeping in for more than nine hours can cause a lot of health problems for you. So, sleep sufficiently and stay fit.

CHAPTER 6

Eat the Right Food

Overeating isn't the only culprit behind your weight gain. Yes, knowing your food and portion control play a key role in helping you maintain your weight (refer to chapter three). There are other aspects to gaining weight, such as eating the wrong stuff and that too at the wrong time. To stay slim and healthy, you need to eat mindfully. You should not just eat anything and get away with it.

Choose your food carefully. Know what's nutritious and what's not good for your body. Don't allow impulse to drive you to eat anything that's available. Yes of course, there could be occasions when you don't have much choice. So, if you have a buffet of different dishes, try and pick stuff that's relatively healthier. For instance, if you have to make a choice between seasonal greens and fried onion tanglers, choose the former.

Keep the thumb rule in mind that whatever you eat should benefit your body in some way. It should not put extra stress on your stomach to digest it. Do a bit of self-talk before you put anything in your mouth—is it good for me, am I going to feel lethargic after having it, is it going to make me feel bloated, or am I taking too many unnecessary calories that I won't be able to shake off.

How to Make Healthy Food Choices

Be vigilant about what you eat. You don't get fat in a day. It takes several cheesy pizzas, hamburgers, cookies, cakes, rolls and butter to make you gain those extra pounds that stay with you like your best friend. It's the food that you choose every single day that makes a difference to your body weight and health.

You have healthy alternatives to everything. Nutritious food doesn't have to be boring. It's your mindset that needs to change to be able to savor healthy food (see chapter one). Without a mind change, you cannot expect a physical change. As soon as you begin to see things in a different light, everything falls into place. Your diet becomes better, you begin to go on regular walks, and you sleep on time every night.

You are the master of your plate. Take charge of it now!

Eat More Fiber

To have a lean body, lean more on fruits, vegetables, and whole grains. They are full of fiber that keeps you full for longer and is packed with many vitamins, antioxidants, and minerals. Fibrous food is low in calories, which means you have no fear of gaining weight. By incorporating more fiber in your meals, you also improve your gut health and avoid constipation.

High-fiber food also helps you stay more energetic, active, and alert. Not to mention the glowing skin that you envy is the work of fiber that helps to keep the body toxins out and give you naturally beautiful skin.

Some of the best high-fiber foods to have are raspberries, blackberries, parsnips, avocado, dried figs, acorn squash, and split peas just to name a few. Besides, try to have water-rich foods, such as watermelon, cucumber, oranges, peaches, celery, tomatoes, grapefruit, and zucchini.

Drink More Water

Make water your favorite drink. Think of it as an alternative to all sorts of beverages that just give you momentary pleasure but nothing long lasting or of value. Water is the most potent drink that helps to keep your system clean. It flushes out the bacteria from your bladder. Make it a habit to drink at least eight to nine glasses of water a day. However, don't gulp it down and get done with it. Always sit and drink water sip by sip.

Drinking more water also helps in keeping your food cravings in check. When you drink a glass of water half an hour before a meal, it prevents you from overeating. Besides, water keeps your body hydrated, which helps you feel more refreshed and calm.

Cut the Sodas

Most of the soda drinks are fun to have not just for their taste but for the fizz as well. However, they are not so healthy and definitely not good for your weight loss plans. They are full of sugar giving you instant kick but lots of calories in the bargain.

Thus, avoid sodas as much as you can. Switch to water and enjoy getting thinner.

Refrain From Having Too Much of Tea or Coffee

Having tea or coffee in a restrained manner, one or two small cups a day, is absolutely fine and it should do you no harm. However, some people are addicted to such beverages. They like to have four to five cups of coffee in a day, which is bad. If you are addicted to caffeine, reduce it to two cups a day.

Avoid milk tea or coffee as much as you can. It's always better to have black tea or coffee without sugar.

Don't Smoke or Have Alcohol

Both smoking and alcohol can have a detrimental impact on your fitness. You may work out every day and eat healthy, but smoking and excessive alcohol can still lead to many lung and heart diseases.

Limit Highly Processed Foods

If you are serious about living a healthy life and staying slim, limit your intake of highly processed foods. In fact, it's better that you completely stay away from foods that have no nutritional value for your body but have plenty of added sugars, saturated fat, and sodium. When you have such foods, your taste buds are happy for a while, but your body suffers in the long run.

Stuff like french fries, burgers, candies, muffins, frozen desserts, and all sorts of processed meats do not get digested so easily. They stay in your intestines long enough to become toxic and contaminate your blood, which makes your body prone to diseases eventually.

Eat Home-Cooked Food

The safest way to eat right is to eat at home. When you cook your own meal, you have complete control over its nutritional value. You can keep the calorie count really low. You can make it a balanced meal with all the right things in place. Home-cooked food can be free of saturated and trans fat. You can make it healthier by adding more seasonal greens, complex carbs, and healthy fats.

Besides, it's a good idea to get creative with your meals. Don't just eat the same stuff every day to get bored. Look up for some new recipes. There's no dearth of healthy recipes that you can easily find online. If you don't eat meat or dairy products, there are so many vegan recipes out there to try. In fact, there are so many healthy dessert recipes for those who have a sweet tooth.

Avoid Fried Food

Deep fried and shallow fried food, both are not as good as they taste. It's better to avoid fried food as much as possible, as they make you feel lethargic and give your body more fat than required. Fried foods make it harder to maintain a healthy body weight.

How to Eat Mindfully

Eating mindfully can change a lot of things for you. The struggle of weight loss will not be a struggle anymore, because you will not gain weight ever in your life. When you eat with awareness, you know what you are eating and why you are eating. You don't eat out of loneliness, boredom, or any emotional reason. You simply eat because you are hungry. The right reason to have food is hunger. You should never eat when you are not hungry.

Get Totally Involved in the Moment of Eating

Allow all your senses to savor food that you eat—listen to the sizzle of hot cooked food, take in the aroma, let your eyes see and appreciate the colors and presentation of food, feel the texture with your hands, and taste the flavors with your tongue. When you soak yourself into the moment of enjoying your food, it's being aware of what you are eating.

Do Not Multitask While Eating

Never eat food with thoughts about other things, such as your work, errands to run, or tasks to finish. Be relaxed when you sit down to have your meal. Don't keep checking your phone every now and then while you are chewing morsels. Keep your phone away. When you eat, just eat. Also, try not to eat alone. It's always better to eat with at least a few people so that you experience the feeling of sharing, partaking in good conversations, and refrain from eating more than you need to.

Eat Slowly

There's nothing better than eating slowly. Most of us gulp down food hurriedly. We are always in a hurry. It's funny but we always forget to chew our food properly, which is also one of the causes of weight gain and various health issues. When you eat your food without chewing, the nutrients are not absorbed by your body to the fullest. Besides, when you eat fast, you end up hogging without realizing when your stomach is full. Therefore, eating slowly makes you chew food properly, take in nutrients, and understand when to stop.

Consider the Food Source

You should also give some thought to the source of food. Think of the farmer who has grown the crop with hard work and given you the privilege to enjoy a meal on your table. Thinking about the food source helps you value food even more and see it in a different light. Instead of thinking of it as something to consume, you respect it and understand its true purpose.

Eat Only When You Are Hungry

You should eat only when your body tells you to eat. Ask yourself, "Am I hungry enough?" Don't just eat for the sake of eating or because you are tempted to eat. Eating when you are hungry helps your body take in food the right way and you feel more satisfied and full.

Respond to Body Signals

If you want to stay lean all your life, listen to your body when it tells you to stop eating. Don't continue to eat even after you feel quite full. In fact, it's even better to stop eating when you feel you still have more scope to eat but you still feel quite appeased. Don't get to the point when you are too full because that leads you toward weight gain.

Benefits of Mindful Eating

Mindful eating can help you in many ways. It's not just good for your body shape or weight, but it's good for your entire being.

Helps You Make Healthier Food Choices

When you eat mindfully, you are able to choose your food more carefully. For instance, if you are invited over by a friend for a meal, you might just get carried away and eat whatever is laid before you. However, mindful eating helps you eat selectively. You may eat more of veggies and less of mashed potatoes from the many things served.

Controls Food Cravings

A mindful eater enjoys their food to the full. They allow each morsel to satiate their appetite, which is why they don't feel any food cravings. You should not eat food because your mind tells you to eat. Food cravings make you overindulge in your favorite food, which often results in the feelings of guilt and regret.

Makes You Eat in a Balanced Way

The best part about eating with awareness is that you eat in a balanced way. Neither do you overeat, nor do you eat less. You are aware of your body, and you feed it with the right stuff—you are conscious about including more colors in your diet—greens, reds, and yellows. Every time you take a meal, you know you are supposed to have more fiber and protein, and less carbs and fats.

Helps in Digestion

When you eat your food properly with no hastiness, a digestive enzyme called amylase is produced in your mouth, which begins the process of digesting carbohydrates. Thus, you should chew your food slowly to enable the enzymes in your digestive tract to break the food down more easily. Poor chewing can cause indigestion, bloating, and gas.

Helps You Enjoy Your Food More

Slow eating or mindful eating also helps you relax and shake off your stress. You are aware that you are eating good food and that makes you enjoy the time. You take pleasure in the taste and flavors, the variety, and the appeal of its appearance.

Keeps You from Overeating

You never overeat when you eat mindfully because you know when to stop. The slow process of mindful eating that involves so much of careful thought and observation helps you eat just the right portion.

Food is necessary for our survival, but it shouldn't rule us. We should enjoy food to the fullest, respect where it's coming from, be aware of its benefits, and eat only as much as we need to.

CHAPTER 7

How to Keep Moving at Home

You don't have to go to a gym or a health club to stay in shape. You can get your body moving within your home as well. You just have to look for ways to do some form of physical exercise whenever you find time. It could be simple squats during commercials or crunches while you are doing the laundry. Cleaning the yard can be a great physical activity, too. The idea is to incorporate physical activities within your domestic realm. Simple habits lead to greater gains.

Some of you might have to spend more time at home than going to work every day. In today's age, when the entire world is connected via technology, you don't have to be physically at work (as long as you are mentally at work). A lot of us have moved to working from home, freelancing, or going to the office occasionally. Besides, you could be a homemaker, a retiree, or someone on a professional break. Well, don't lie on the sofa eating peanuts. Stop being lazy. Get up and move your body.

When you don't move your body, you get into trouble. It's quite simple! It's not just about gaining weight. When you sit too much watching TV or working on your laptop, you get problems like pain in your back, shoulders, or legs, and also fatigue, stress, and digestive issues.

Thus, embrace home workouts to stay lean and keep your body devoid of diseases. Let's check out some of the simplest of physical activities that you can do without going out. And remember, staying physically active is fun and stress-relieving. It's not something cumbersome or boring.

Get Involved in Household Chores

When you are home, there's so much to do. Depending on whether you stay alone or with family, you can get involved in various household chores. You don't have to take up everything and feel burnt out. Choose your favorite stuff to do. For instance, you might like vacuum cleaning. Take the vacuum cleaner and clean up everything. While it may not be a great workout, it will definitely prevent you from sitting.

You should think of ways to make your household chores fun and easy. For instance, you may enjoy cooking a meal while listening to a nice podcast. You could also think of ways to get creative with your housework—whether it's putting dishes in the dishwasher or clothes in the washing machine, just look for ways to move your body a little bit more. You can do some heel raises while doing the chores. Get more precise with whatever you do, like segregating your clothes before washing them, arranging dishes in a different way, or preparing the dining table before each meal.

Exercise While You Are Still in Bed

If you are not a morning person, fret not. You can exercise as soon as you wake up right where you are—in your bed. Yes, there are quite a few exercises that can be easily done in a bed, such as leg marches, reverse crunches, straight leg lifts, and handstand push-ups to name a few. These exercises are good for toning your hips, abs, and shoulders.

As you finish your bed exercises, be sure to make your own bed. Folding bed sheets, arranging pillows, and pulling up bed covers can be a bit of a physical activity. It requires you to use your hand muscles quite a bit as some bed sheets are heavy to fold. The small bits at home help you stay in shape.

Keep Walking

There's nothing easier than to walk (refer chapter four). So, keep walking within your home as well. You may be sitting on a chair for some time, get up after 15-20 minutes and get moving. Go to the refrigerator (not to pick up some dessert) and get some lemon to squeeze into a glass of water. Walk toward your favorite window of the house from where you can possibly catch a nice view outside. If there's no view, simply stand there for some fresh air. Never sit and take phone calls. Always try to walk while on calls. That's also a good excuse to be walking.

You can also split your half an hour walk into three 10-minute walks thrice in a day. You can walk for 10 minutes in the morning, another 10 minutes anytime of the day, and the last 10 minutes post dinner.

Dance to Elevate Your Mood

You should spend some time dancing to some upbeat tune, at least once in a while. Dance isn't just an exercise, but it's an excellent way to uplift your mood, keep your stress level low, and keep the blood in your veins flowing. Don't worry even if you don't know how to dance. These days you have access to many online dance classes. Perhaps you could join one of them. The best part about dancing is that it doesn't feel like a workout. You sweat it out with joy.

Set Reminders to Avoid Sitting Around for Long

You can set reminder alarms on your phone to nudge you to stand up and do something every 30 minutes. For instance, if you work 9 to 12 in the first half of the day, you can take a 10 minute breather a couple of times, or more. Just stand and move around, grab a glass of water or stretch a little bit. You can also set reminders for your favorite activities like reading, playing a musical instrument, or talking to a friend. Well, reading may involve sitting or reclining. But you can refrain from doing so. Instead, spend some time standing at the bookcase to pick and choose a book. Besides, you can always walk and read.

Climb the Stairs

You should climb the stairs every day without fail. It's the best way to burn calories (even better than walking). It's an effective, low-impact cardio exercise. If you have the option of climbing stairs in your home, make it one of your must-do activities every day. Whenever you want to take a break from work or you just want to shake off the lethargy, take the stairs. Climbing stairs keeps your leg and hip muscles in shape besides toning your abdominal muscles.

Stretch and Breathe Whenever You Have Time

Stretching your body from head to toe every now and then is also an effective way of staying active. As you stretch your limbs and straighten your back, make sure to breathe in and out as well. Combining your breathing exercises with stretching can work wonders. It's a good way to keep your body in shape, especially the back and abdominal. Not to mention it releases stress from your shoulders and neck.

Use TV Time to Work Out

We spend long hours watching TV or Netflix, mostly munching away our favorite snack or opening a soda bottle. Well, there's no harm in doing that once in a while. However, you should refrain from lazing around too often. Make it a point to use your movie time for some crunches or squats. While you are on the sofa for half an hour, get up to work out for at least 15-20 minutes and then again relax for some time. If you sit down to watch TV for 45-60 minutes, make sure to stand up and do some physical activity for at least 20 minutes.

Run After Your Kids or Pets

If you have kids or pets, they are sure to keep you quite busy with a lot of running around. So, you should enjoy it to the fullest. The more you run after them, the more calories you lose. Think of different ways to engage with them, so that the time you spend with them becomes more rewarding and fun. For instance, you can play outdoor sports with your kids or make them clean their room.

You can take your dog for a walk, which is a great physical as well as mental activity for you.

Spend Time Gardening

Gardening is also a good way to keep yourself physically occupied. In fact, there's quite a lot of manual work involved in gardening—digging, lifting pots, walking, and mowing the lawn. Besides, you also want to rearrange different pots, which requires you to move around. You can burn up to 200-300 calories by just working in your garden. Not to mention it can also take away a lot of mental stress and refresh you.

Although gardening is definitely a great way to stay active, it may not help everyone to lose significant weight. We all have different bodies with different metabolisms. Thus, some people require more hardcore exercises and a specific diet plan to burn fat. You shouldn't just depend on gardening to get into shape.

Set Aside Time for Your Favorite Exercise

If you are home most of the time, you can easily manage time for some sort of physical exercise—it could be yoga, crunches, squats, pushups, lunges, hip rotations, planks, leg raises, or Pilates. You don't need any gym equipment to lose weight or stay fit. You will have to be mentally firm about dedicating at least 30-45 minutes to physical workout at least four times a week. It could be in the morning or in the evening. You can choose your time according to your work schedule and household chores.

To motivate yourself, you can workout with a partner instead of doing it alone. It's more fun to workout with somebody. You can also keep a journal to give yourself goals and note down your progress. Keep a playlist ready and get on your exercise mat!

Whether you stay home or go out for work, be intentional about incorporating a lot of physical activities in a normal day. Don't wait for the weekends or for some special days when you will get time to exercise. Being physically active should be the constant thing in your life.

CHAPTER 8

Diet and Exercise Myths

Don't fall prey to fitness myths. In today's age, everybody has an opinion about diets and exercises. Some will tell you to abstain from certain foods to lose weight while some will advise you to work out for two hours. Perhaps fitness is one of the most debatable topics today. Many blogs and articles have been written about staying lean. So many food brands have catered toward the needs of fitness freaks. And yes, we have weight loss coaches and fitness apps available on our smartphones.

There are all sorts of diets for you to choose from—the paleo diet, the vegan diet, low-carb diets, the low-fat diet, and the ketogenic diet. It's normal for anyone to get confused about what to choose. Well, you should just relax. When there are too many ideas and opinions floating around, you should apply your own common sense. Each individual has the ability to decide the best fitness regime for themselves. The first thing you should understand is that everyone is different. Although the basic guideline for good health and fitness is the same for everyone, there are quite a few variations in terms of diets and exercises for different people.

To understand and decide what's ideal for you in regards to weight management, you should consider certain factors like your age, environment, and your staple food. If you live in a hot place, you will have certain foods while also refrain from having certain foods. For instance, people who live in coastal regions will have coconut water because that's easily available to them. Common sense should tell you to eat what's locally available, and also what's seasonal. If you eat something that's been in cold storage for six months until it reaches your plate, it's not going to give much nutrition to your body.

Thus, what to eat and what not to eat should largely depend on where you live and how active you are physically. Perhaps you can have meat every day as long as you are young and work out four times a week. However, if you have advanced in years and live a pretty sedentary life, there's no point taking in much fat. So besides choosing local and seasonal food, you should consider your age and lifestyle when it comes to choosing what to eat to stay lean and healthy.

You should not eat something just because it's been recommended by a few experts. Make it a point to think from a holistic perspective—consider factors like its availability, freshness, and sustainability. If you eat something that's marked as "super healthy", but it's sourced and packed in some distant place, from where it takes miles to get to a store near you, the so-called nutritional value of the product is not worth it. Instead of having something that isn't produced regionally or is not in season, it's better to have something which is locally produced and is in season.

Whether you are struggling to come out of obesity or trying to maintain a healthy weight, myths and facts are going to surround you. Take some time and do your own research, understand your own body, and follow a sensible fitness regime. The basic idea is to follow something that's traditional and good—for example, you should have breakfast in the morning. Don't go after new ideologies without some thought, common sense, and research.

Let's bust some fitness myths here—

You Can Eat Anything if You Exercise

Unfortunately, there's no substitute to a good diet. If you think you can eat whatever you feel like as long as you sweat it out, that's not going to work. A fit body is a combination of a good diet and a sensible workout regime. You cannot have good health and fitness with an imbalanced diet no matter how much you exercise. You need to have correct portions of all nutrients that you get from carbs, proteins, and fat. When you do any kind of physical exercise regularly, it helps your body utilize nutrients in a proper way. The calories that you take are not stored as fat but converted into energy. Protein helps your body to build muscles. Carbs give your body the required strength. So each has its own role to play in your diet.

Thus, you need to have a balanced diet every day. You cannot take calories or fat mindlessly just because you can burn it out in the gym. You might be able to stay thin by sweating it out a bit extra, but it's not going to keep your body healthy in the long run. Besides, the research says that your weight loss depends on 70% of what you eat and 30% of how much you exercise. So, you definitely need to watch what you eat.

Walking Is Not a Workout

Well, we have a chapter dedicated to walking and how it can help you stay fit (refer chapter 4). Walking is a great workout. In fact, it gets your whole body into movement. A brisk walk helps you sweat out—makes your heart race faster, your lungs breathe more, the blood flow increases, and you burn a lot of calories. Walking is suitable for all age groups. Perhaps walking isn't considered a serious workout by many because it doesn't involve any equipment or difficulty level. But it doesn't have to. Anything that helps you shed some calories and keeps your weight in control is a workout.

You Should Feel Pain Post Workout

Many believe that physical exercise should hurt. It should make your body sore. Well, that's not necessary at all. Of course, when you begin to exercise or workout after a long time, your body does ache. However, it's completely pointless to make your body suffer in the name of exercise. In fact, working out should be a pleasant experience. Yes, you should push your body, allow it to build its stamina. But you need to do it slowly. You should never push your body beyond a point. It's not going to make weight loss faster for you. Worse, you are more likely to miss out on your workouts because of pain and injuries.

You Need to Have Perfect Weight and

Waistline

It's good to be lean and fit; however, it's not quite good to be obsessed with perfection. Not all healthy and fit people have the same body weights and waistlines. An ideal body weight or waistline is quite subjective. Yes of course, your body weight should be in proportion to your height. However, it can vary from person to person according to their age, metabolism, and other factors.

Besides, a perfect weight and waistline doesn't mean perfect health. A person with a not-so-perfect waistline can also be healthy and have a strong immune system. You might want to go crazy after six pack abs, but they don't guarantee great inner strength. So, don't overstress yourself with the idea of a perfect body. Go after strength, immunity, and fitness.

Supplements Can Help You Become Lean

It's a big trap that you can get into. No supplement can ever make you lose weight. Don't fall for the marketing tactics of many companies who just try to sell their products. The truth is that most supplements are ineffective in helping you become slim. Even if you do get lean, it's not worth the investment as it's not the genuine way of getting into shape. We get to the basics again, which is to focus on a wholesome life of good food, good exercise, and good sleep. When you combine all three in a balanced way, you don't need any quick fixes or artificial ways of slimming down.

Eating Multiple Times is Not Good

There are people who eat less thinking they will stay lean that way. On the contrary, you can have multiple meals in a day and still stay slim. Some people like to eat three times a day—breakfast, lunch, and dinner. They don't like to snack between meals, which is fine. However, there's another way to plan your meals, which is to eat five times a day—breakfast, midday meal, lunch, afternoon tea, and dinner. There's no harm in having five to six meals in a day. It will not make you fat or prevent you from shedding weight. Eating multiple times doesn't mean snacking on chocolates or chips. As long as you eat healthy and in a balanced way, you will be fine.

You Should Stop Having Carbs to Lose Weight

Perhaps this is one of the most popular myths out there and it needs to be busted hard. You should never stop having carbs, not even think of going on a low-carb diet. That's not a very sustainable way of shedding weight. You might lose weight pretty quick, but you will lose a lot of other things along the way. Since carbs give you energy and many micronutrients to stay healthy, you cannot live without them for long.

The adverse effects of carb deprivation could be slow metabolism, fatigue, dehydration, and muscle ache. You should not give up something which is foundational for your body. You cannot live on a low-carb or no carb diet all your life. Thus, it's better to never get on such diets in the first place. Instead, opt for portion control, which we have discussed in chapter three.

All Fat is Bad

Fat is such a bad word. But is it really bad? Well, not all fat is bad for your health (refer chapter 3). There are good fats as well—unsaturated fats—monounsaturated and polyunsaturated fats that reduce the risk of diseases in your body. You should take good fats through stuff like whole eggs, fish, nuts, olive oil, and avocados. Throwing away the yolk of an egg and having only the white is not the healthiest thing to do—the yolk has many essential minerals and vitamins; and no, it doesn't let your cholesterol increase. Yes, excess of anything is not advisable. You can safely have one whole egg a day and be just fine.

Good fats support cell growth in your body, help you absorb vitamins, aid in brain and eye health, and keep you energetic. So, include healthy fats in your daily diet.

You Should Avoid Sugar Totally

Yes, refined sugar is not good for your body. However, don't eliminate sugar completely from your diet. Remember, there are many forms of natural sugar, such as honey, jaggery, and dates which are quite healthy. Besides, there are quite a few high-sugar fruits, such as mangoes, cherries, pears, watermelons, figs, and bananas which you should have.

Also, there's no harm in enjoying your favorite dessert once in a while (even if it's made with white sugar). It's not going to make you fat or unhealthy. Neither you gain weight in a day nor you lose weight in a day. It's what you do consistently that makes you who you are. Don't be afraid to sweeten it up whenever you need to.

Skipping Meals Helps You Lose Weight Faster

You should have all your meals on time. It's what you eat and how much you eat that makes you thin or fat. Skipping meals is not a solution to weight gain. Intermittent fasting is a different idea, which we have covered in chapter three. However, not having breakfast or any meal for that matter with an idea of slimming down is not good. You will lose muscle mass and not burn fat by not eating. There's nothing like fast weight loss anyway. Weight loss has to be combined with eating and exercising sensibly.

If you want to lose weight sustainably, make sure to have all your meals along with regular workouts.

You Should Count Each Calorie That You Take

It's not a good idea to go insane for the sake of losing weight. Counting each calorie is not practical and it's not even good for your mental health. You should eat what you need to eat. It's a practice that you need to stick to and make it a habit—that you don't overeat or eat for emotional reasons. You can eat junk food once in a while, but then you will have to understand how often that 'once in a while' is going to happen. If you can keep yourself from eating junk completely, nothing like it.

You don't need to count calories. All you have to ensure, which you will understand with time, is that you shouldn't consume more calories than you are able to use. For instance, if your job doesn't require you to move around much and you walk for about 20-30 minutes a day, you should take calories accordingly. Don't go overboard because you know you cannot burn the extra calories. However, you shouldn't consume more calories just because you workout more.

Men and Women Need Different Exercises

People assume that men should be lifting heavy weights and women should be on the yoga mat. Gender is not the factor when it comes to the kind of exercises one needs. Men and women may be different in many ways, but they need the same exercises to stay fit. Some believe that strength training or weight training is not for women, which is far from the truth. In fact, as you age, your muscle mass depletes, and bones begin to degenerate. Therefore, it's even more necessary to strengthen your muscles by some weight training.

You Should Work Out Every Day

Some people believe the more you work out, the leaner you get. But that's not the right approach to fitness. You should have your rest days. You can choose to work out five days a week, four days a week, or even three days a week. It's totally up to you. Exercising every day or sweating it out in the gym for longer than usual is not going to make you fitter than anyone else. You need to have a balanced approach toward your workouts as well. If you work out too much, it will make you feel burnt out after a while. The idea behind taking a break of a day or two is to give your body time to rest and refresh. Working out for half an hour to 45 minutes four to five times a week is sufficient for most people.

Health and fitness need to be tackled with wisdom. You shouldn't just go after what's popular and trending. You have the ability to judge and understand what's right for you. The key is to understand everything scientifically and logically.

CHAPTER 9

Gear Up for the Day

The right start to anything can make a big difference to how it's going to flow ahead. Starting your day right is the key to a lot of good things in life, including a fit body. You should wake up with an anticipation in your heart for something good to happen. Be intentional about your day. Take charge of your will and action. Plan in your head how you are going to spend the day.

Smart people don't go with the flow. They are purposeful and decisive. They know what they want and what they don't want. They are not afraid to eliminate things from their schedule. People who aspire to live a wholesome life always do things for their own betterment. They live consciously. They are aware of their surroundings, their strengths, and also their limitations. People who have progressive mindsets don't mull over their failures or weaknesses too much—they mull over only to learn something out of it. They believe in looking ahead and doing the best for themselves and also for others around them.

People who appear lean, fit, and healthy invest their efforts into good things. They set their priorities right. They know how to choose the right things amongst the many options available—they choose waking up early over late-nights, walking over taking a bus, eating fresh locally-produced vegetables over some exotic pizza, and staying positive over staying negative. We get choices every day. It's the simple things that we do every day that lead us to greater successes in life.

To stay lean and maintain a steady body weight, you don't have to do something crazy for a few days and just get done with it. You don't have to live on pills or on some health juices. All you have to do is live a healthy, balanced life. As we head toward the end of the book, you must have understood that weight loss cannot be a short-term goal. It's something that you need to follow all your life, in a way that it becomes a lifestyle.

How to Start Your Day Right

You should be particular about how you want to start your day. In fact, you should look forward to waking up every morning. There are people who wake up with the help of an alarm clock, and then there are those who like to keep hitting the snooze button until it's too late and they have no choice but to get out of bed. Well, it's okay if you want to be that way as long as you don't feel guilty about it. The point to deal with is that most of us struggle to do the right thing and we constantly feel grouchy about it.

The earlier you get out of bed, the better it is because then you have more time to do a lot of things that you want to do, such as going for a walk, getting most of the office work done, learning a new skill, or just enjoying time doing nothing. To live a quality life, it's important to spend some time doing nothing. Being always busy and stressed out isn't defined as a very successful life. A holistic living is about making use of your time wisely, which should include everything—your daily tasks, workouts, office, meeting people, eating meals, spending time with family, listening to music, watching a movie, reading a book, meditating, relaxing, and sleeping. You live a successful life when you find time to do everything. Of course, there will be days when you will be excessively busy with work or occupied with personal commitments, and you will miss out on relaxing or going for a walk. The idea is to have a plan in your mind about your day.

Decide How You Want to Spend the First Hour of Your Day

Ideally, the first thing you should do in the morning is to check your "to-do" sort of a list, which should inspire you to have an exciting start of the day. Grab a glass of water, flush the toxins out, and feel refreshed. Set out to take in some fresh air and walk a mile. Come back and catch up on the news, check your phone (yes, you may do that after you have done a few meaningful things), and have some fresh fruits. Your breakfast time should be leisurely and enjoyable. You shouldn't rush through it. Sit down to have breakfast. Use the breakfast time to connect with your spouse and children, or whoever you are living with.

Savor Every Bit of Your Morning

It's extremely important to savor your morning time. It's the most precious time of the day because both your mind and body are fresh. Morning is the best time to start something new—it could be writing a book, playing a sport, or practicing a skill. It's the most productive time of the day. You can accomplish a lot in the first few hours of the morning.

Being aware of the power of morning hours, you can achieve your weight loss goals with much ease. If you spend your morning hours sleeping, the rest of the day is not going to reward you as much. Of course, you can get lean even when you get up late. There's no rule for weight loss. People lose weight in many ways. However, the best way to make fitness a lifestyle for you, waking up early and getting into a physical activity that you enjoy is quite helpful.

Follow a Morning Ritual

Your morning should be about activities that connect you to something meaningful and long-lasting—things you know in your heart that they are good for you. It could be praying, working in your yard, talking to your children or someone who you look up to, writing a gratitude journal, practicing yoga, or just sitting quietly observing your surroundings. Just do whatever you truly enjoy every morning without fail. Make it a ritual.

How to Plan Your Day

Planning your day helps you spend it right. When you just wake up and start your day without any awareness or purpose, your mind doesn't support your goals. You think about doing something, but you never get to the point of doing it. That's when you feel frustrated and clueless. Losing weight and keeping it off doesn't happen with random plans. It doesn't happen with a mere thought or a random day of hardcore workout. It takes planning and determination in your mind. Therefore, it's important to plan your day.

Make a To-Do List

Every night as you go to bed, keep your diary and pen on your side table and jot down what you will be doing the next day. As you wake up the next morning, look at the list of things to be ticked off. Get done with the most difficult task first and leave the easy ones for the later part of the day. For instance, you should do your half an hour of cardio workout within the first few hours of the morning. Keep activities like going out, shopping, or meeting a friend for later.

Your to-do list should be built around your goals. If you aim to lose 10 pounds in four to six months, make sure some sort of physical activity is part of your daily routine. Besides, you need to ensure you eat right and keep certain things off your plate if not your kitchen. You will have to stop eating high-sugar stuff like chocolates, ice creams, cold coffee, cakes, cookies, and all sorts of desserts; and also high-fat stuff like pizzas, butter, cheese, cream, and bacon. You will have to pick more vegetables, fruits, nuts, whole grains, and lean meat. To do that, you will need to plan your food shopping.

Keep Your To-Do List Realistic

It's always more helpful to have a mix of both short-term and long-term goals on your to-do list. Don't have too many things planned in a day. Keep it at five things to be ticked off in a day. Make sure you are able to accomplish at least three from the list every day, and the rest two can be done within a week or two. For instance, you should be going for a walk and eating vegetables every day; however, you can procrastinate grocery shopping or decluttering the wardrobe. Procrastination isn't always bad as long as you have programmed your mind well and you live your life in a structured way.

Focus to Finish One Task a Day

The ideal way to get most of the things done is to simply focus on one big task a day. When we try to accomplish a lot in a day, we end up doing nothing substantial. We appear busy but we are barely productive. However, when you aim to get done with one big task in a day, that gives you the energy to get done with other smaller tasks as well. So, when you look at it on a weekly basis, you will be happy to realize you have accomplished five to seven big things in a week.

For instance, you can focus on drinking more water and cutting down on caffeine on Monday, walk for an hour on Tuesday, go for a dance class on Wednesday, eat only fruits and vegetables on Thursday (it could be a great way to try intermittent fasting), clean up your yard on Friday, and pair up with somebody for a cardio session on Saturday. You can keep Sundays relaxed and aimless. Perhaps you can reward yourself with a scoop of your favorite ice cream with a cherry on top.

Plan to Subdue Your Cravings

Have a plan to deal with the inevitable, which is your craving to snack on something during the day. If you have nothing at hand, you will end up snacking on whatever is available. You don't want to snack on potato chips or pringles when you have had an hour-long workout session in the morning. Thus, it's nice to pack some healthy snacks to munch. For instance, you can have a carrot, an apple, some nuts, or wholegrain crackers whenever you feel the urge.

Set Apart Time for a Little Workout Before Lunch

Well, if you are not a morning person and trying too hard to shed some weight, plan to workout for 30 minutes before lunch. It's the lean hour of the day, which will allow you to exercise without a distraction. Besides, you will gain more energy to carry on with the rest of the day. Perhaps you will also be able to skip that afternoon coffee.

You should have a protein rich meal post workout, which will help your body build muscles and lose weight faster.

Plan to Spend Some Time Outdoors

The easiest way to move your body is to spend some time outdoors—relaxing on the grass, reading a book under a tree, swimming, playing, walking or running in a park, visiting a farm or a vineyard, or simply walking the street. Spending time outdoors is necessary for your mental health as well, because there's no better nurturer and healer than nature. Not to mention you need sunshine and fresh air, too.

Plan to Relax in the Evenings

After a hectic day, plan to have a relaxed evening. You should do something completely different from what you have done the entire day. For instance, if you have racked your brain too much at work, don't sit down to read a book. Instead, play with your dog and spend time with your family. Alternatively, you can also get into an elaborative cooking session with some nice music in the background.

Starting your day right and planning each day can make a huge difference to your lifestyle. You will see the benefits in the long run and the benefits are going to last. You will know the key to healthy living because you will have mastered it.

Conclusion

Now is the time to get started with your own fitness journey. It's not too late yet. You can lose weight without starving or dieting. In fact, you should enjoy eating without guilt because now you know how to eat mindfully and how to choose the right food. You have the power to rule your mind. You know your body. You understand its needs. You have learned portion control. You don't need motivation to get into a physical fitness regime because you know how to enjoy going on regular walks and staying active all day. You have learned the art of creating a sleep routine. You know how to start your day right.

With this book, you have got the kick to live holistically with new habits and behaviors. The right approach to physical fitness is to focus on your overall well-being and not just on getting a narrow waistline. Being healthy is about being in control of your thoughts and actions. It's about following a certain lifestyle. When you know the right thing to do and you have the right approach to do it too, nothing is too hard to achieve. Most people know what to do but they never get to do it because they don't know the right approach to it.

You don't have to suffer to be able to get rid of your extra weight and to keep it off. It's a mindset change, which enables you to change your ways. You let go of certain food habits and in exchange, you adapt to some new food habits. So, you don't really miss out on anything. Life should be about constant changes, improvements, and upliftments. Think of weight loss as something meant to give you more happiness and satisfaction in the long run. Thus, don't let it become a short-term goal. Learn to enjoy it. Embrace the idea of exercising every day. Take pleasure in picking and choosing your food. Give yourself new challenges. Eat right and exercise with the end goal feeling in mind. When you know the reward is something extraordinary, you don't mind stretching yourself a little extra. There's nothing that comes without some effort.

Focus on being consistent with small things. Don't overwhelm yourself with ideologies like depriving yourself of carbs or working hard in the gym to get six pack abs. You don't have to do all that. Keep it simple, easy, and consistent. The key is to be persistent and not be enslaved by misconceptions and laziness.

Let the three core things take precedence in your daily routine—nutritious food, physical exercise, and a definite bedtime. As you incorporate simple changes in your daily life, you will soon realize it wasn't too hard and staying lean is all about doing the basics right. Take action today!

References

Beck, L. (2018, June 1). Why weighing your food can make a difference for your health. *The Globe and Mail.* https://www.theglobeandmail.com/life/health-and-fitness/article-why-weighing-your-food-can-make-a-difference-for-your-health/

Ellis, E. (2018). *Eating Right Isn't Complicated.* Eatright.org. https://www.eatright.org/food/nutrition/dietary-guidelines-and-myplate/eating-right-isnt-complicated

Fry, A. (2020, September 11). *Why Do We Need Sleep?* Sleep Foundation. https://www.sleepfoundation.org/how-sleep-works/why-do-we-need-sleep

Hare, H. V. (2017, October 27). *25 food and exercise myths everyone should stop believing*. Insider. https://www.insider.com/food-and-exercise-myths-2017-10

John Hopkins Medicine. (2021). *Intermittent Fasting: What is it, and how does it work?* Www.hopkinsmedicine.org. https://www.hopkinsmedicine.org/health/wellness-and-prevention/intermittent-fasting-what-is-it-and-how-does-it-work

Mayo Clinic. (2017). *Can you boost your metabolism?* Mayo Clinic. https://www.mayoclinic.org/healthy-lifestyle/weight-loss/in-depth/metabolism/art-20046508

Ph.D, S. C. C. (2015, November 3). *The Boomerang Effect: How lost weight finds its way home.*

Https://Www.inquirer.com. https://www.inquirer.com/philly/blogs/goal-getter-nutrition/The-Boomerang-Effect-How-lost-weight-finds-its-way-home.html

Rabbitt, M. (2018, May 8). *10 Amazing Health Benefits of Walking 30 Minutes a Day, According to Doctors.* Prevention; Prevention. https://www.prevention.com/fitness/a20485587/benefits-from-walking-every-day/

Robinson, L. (n.d.). *Mindful Eating - HelpGuide.org.* Https://Www.helpguide.org. https://www.helpguide.org/articles/diets/mindful-eating.htm#

September 7, J. C., & 2020. (2020, September 7). *6 Mindset Changes That Help You Lose Weight Fast.* Eat This Not That. https://www.eatthis.com/mindset-changes-lose-weight/

Zelman, K. M., MPH, RD, & LD. (n.d.). *8 Ways to Think Thin.* WebMD. https://www.webmd.com/diet/obesity/features/8-ways-to-think-thin#1

Made in the USA
Monee, IL
04 November 2026

67387468R00056